I0704603

Delicious
Diabetic-Friendly Recipes

A Cookbook for Managing Diabetes and Enjoying Great Food

Dr. Victoria Holly

All rights reserved. No part of this publication may be reproduced, distributed, or transmitted in any form or by any means, including photocopying, recording, or other electronic or mechanical methods, without the prior written permission of the publisher, except in the case of brief quotations embodied in critical reviews and certain other non-commercial uses permitted by copyright law.

Copyright © Dr. Victoria Holly, 2023.

TABLE OF CONTENT

An introduction to diabetes and how it affects nutrition

Diabetes

Diabetes is a chronic disease that affects millions of people around the world. It occurs when the body is unable to properly process and use insulin, a hormone that regulates blood sugar levels. There are two main types of diabetes: type 1 and type 2.

Type 1 diabetes, also known as juvenile diabetes, is an autoimmune disorder in which the body's immune system attacks and destroys the cells in the pancreas that produce insulin. As a result, people with type 1 diabetes must take insulin injections or use an insulin pump to manage their blood sugar levels.

Type 2 diabetes, on the other hand, is caused by a combination of factors, including genetics, obesity, and a sedentary lifestyle. In type 2 diabetes, the body either doesn't produce enough insulin or the cells in the body become resistant to it. This leads to a build-up of sugar in the bloodstream, which can cause serious health problems if left untreated.

Symptoms of diabetes can include increased thirst and urination, fatigue, blurred vision, and slow wound healing. People with type 2 diabetes may also experience numbness or tingling in their feet. If you suspect you may have diabetes, it's important to see a healthcare provider for a blood sugar test.

Managing diabetes requires a combination of healthy eating, regular physical activity, and medications or insulin therapy as needed. A diet that is rich in fruits, vegetables, whole grains, and lean protein, along with regular physical activity, can help manage blood sugar levels and reduce the risk of complications.

People with diabetes also need to monitor their blood sugar levels regularly and work closely with a healthcare provider to adjust their treatment plan as needed. This may involve taking medication or insulin, monitoring blood sugar levels, and making changes to diet and exercise.

While diabetes can be a challenging condition to manage, with the right treatment and lifestyle changes, people with diabetes can lead long and healthy lives. It's important to take an active role in managing your diabetes, working closely with your healthcare provider, and making healthy lifestyle choices to help keep blood sugar levels under control.

If you're newly diagnosed or are looking for ways to manage your diabetes, don't hesitate to reach out to your healthcare provider, they can help provide guidance and support as you navigate this condition. There are also a lot of online resources and support groups available, which can be a helpful source of information and emotional support for people with diabetes and their loved ones.

Diabetes can greatly affect a person's nutrition, as the disease affects the body's ability to process and use sugar, which is a major source of energy for the body. In order to maintain healthy blood sugar levels, people with diabetes need to pay close attention to their diet and make certain adjustments.

One of the most important aspects of diabetes nutrition is carbohydrate management. Carbohydrates are broken down into glucose (sugar) by the body and raise blood sugar levels, so people with diabetes need to be mindful of the amount and type of carbohydrates they consume. This can include counting carbohydrates, following a meal plan that is low in carbohydrates, and choosing carbohydrates that are high in fiber and low on the glycemic index.

Protein and fats also play a role in diabetes nutrition. It's important for people with diabetes to choose lean proteins such as fish, chicken, and legumes and to limit their intake of saturated fats found in red meat and butter. Replacing saturated fats with healthy fats such as olive oil and avocado can help keep cholesterol levels in check.

A healthy diet for people with diabetes should also be rich in fruits, vegetables, and whole grains. These foods are high in essential vitamins, minerals, and fiber, and they are also low in calories and carbohydrates.

In addition to a healthy diet, regular physical activity is also crucial for managing diabetes. Exercise helps to lower blood sugar levels by moving glucose out of the blood and into the muscles, where it can be used as energy.

It is also important to mention that monitoring blood sugar levels regularly and taking medications as prescribed by a healthcare professional can also greatly help in managing diabetes.

Overall, diabetes affects nutrition by requiring a person to be more mindful of their food choices, portion sizes, and overall meal planning. However, with the help of a registered dietitian or a nutritionist, it is possible to create a personalized meal plan that meets an individual's specific needs and preferences.

There are several key nutrients that can help to manage blood sugar levels in the body. Some of these include:

Fiber: Soluble fiber, in particular, can slow down the absorption of sugar in the gut, which can help to keep blood sugar levels stable. Good sources of soluble fiber include oats, barley, legumes, and some fruits and vegetables.

Chromium: This mineral helps to improve insulin sensitivity and can help to regulate blood sugar levels. Chromium can be found in foods like broccoli, grape juice, and egg yolks.

Magnesium: Low levels of magnesium are associated with insulin resistance, and getting enough of this mineral can help to improve insulin sensitivity and regulate blood sugar levels. Good sources of magnesium include leafy greens, nuts, and seeds.

Alpha-lipoic acid: This antioxidant can help to improve insulin sensitivity and lower blood sugar levels. It can be found in foods such as spinach, broccoli, and potatoes.

Cinnamon: This spice has been found to have blood sugar-lowering effects by helping to improve insulin sensitivity.

Alpha-glucosidase inhibitors : Some of the natural alpha-glucosidase inhibitors like Acarbose and miglitol can help in delaying the absorption of carbohydrates in the gut, thus slowing down the spike in blood sugar level after a meal.

It's important to note that while these nutrients can be beneficial, they should not be used as a substitute for medical treatment or lifestyle changes that are recommended by a healthcare professional. A healthy diet, regular exercise, and maintaining a healthy weight are all important factors in managing blood sugar levels.

It's always best to consult with a healthcare professional or a dietitian for personalized advice on managing blood sugar levels and be sure to check for any possible interactions with any medications you are currently taking.

Tips for eating out and navigating restaurant menus when you have diabetes.

Eating out at a restaurant can be challenging for people with diabetes, as it can be difficult to know the nutritional content of the food and how it will affect blood sugar levels.

Here are a few tips for eating out and navigating restaurant menus when you have diabetes:

1. **Plan ahead:** Before going to a restaurant, take a look at the menu online and plan ahead what you are going to order. This can help you make a more informed decision and avoid impulsively ordering something that may not be as healthy.

2. **Ask questions:** Don't be afraid to ask your server or the chef about the ingredients and preparation methods of the dishes. Ask for

modifications, like requesting to have your dish made with less oil or sugar.

3. **Watch portion sizes:** Restaurant portions are often much larger than what is recommended for people with diabetes. Share an entree with a friend, or ask the server to pack half of your meal to take home for later.

4. **Watch for hidden sugar:** Many restaurant dishes contain added sugar, so be wary of items such as sauces, marinades, and salad dressings, which can be high in sugar.

5. **Opt for lean protein:** Choose dishes that are high in protein and low in saturated fat, such as grilled chicken, fish, or tofu.

6. **Add non-starchy vegetables:** Balance your meal with a big salad or side of non-starchy vegetables like spinach, broccoli, or bell peppers.

7. **Specialty Diet option:** Many restaurants today offer options for those who have a special dietary needs and preferences such as gluten-free, low carb, diabetic-friendly, etc. If a restaurant has such options, take advantage of it!

8. **Be mindful of alcohol intake:** Alcohol can affect blood sugar levels, so limit alcohol consumption and opt for drinks that are lower in carbohydrates, such as wine or light beer.

Keep in mind that with any dietary changes, it's important to consult with a healthcare professional or a registered dietitian for personalized advice.

Additionally, eating out will require extra attention and self-control, but with the right mindset and preparation, it is possible to have a good time and still maintain your health goals.

Meal planning and prepping, including tips for keeping your kitchen stocked with healthy ingredients, and how to make the most of leftovers.

Meal planning and prepping can be an effective way to manage blood sugar levels and stay on track with a healthy diet when you have diabetes.

Here are a few suggestions for meal planning and prepping:

- **Plan your meals for the week:** Take some time each week to plan out your meals for the upcoming days. This can help you make sure that you have the ingredients you need on hand, and it can also help you make healthier choices.

- **Make a grocery list:** Once you've planned your meals, make a grocery list of the ingredients you'll need. This can help you avoid buying unnecessary items and can also help you stick to your budget.

- **Cook in bulk:** Cooking in bulk can save time and money. Make extra servings of your meals and freeze them for later, or make large batches of healthy meals that can be easily reheated throughout the week.

- **Keep it simple**: Simple meals are often the easiest to prepare and can be just as nutritious as more complex dishes. Focus on using whole, nutrient-dense ingredients, and keep seasonings and flavors simple.

- **Use the right storage containers:** Invest in good quality, airtight storage containers that are suitable for keeping food fresh. This will make it easier to store and keep food fresh for longer periods of time.

- **Make use of leftovers:** Instead of letting leftovers go to waste, make use of them as part of your meal plan, this will save time and money.

- **Have a balanced plan:** Make sure your meals have a balance of carbohydrates, proteins, and healthy fats. This can help keep blood sugar levels stable, and also make sure you have enough energy throughout the day.

- **Be open to experimenting with new recipe**: Having a diverse range of meal options can help prevent boredom and make sticking to a meal plan more manageable.

Consulting with a registered dietitian is always helpful when planning and prepping meals. They can provide personalized guidance on how to structure your meals, what foods are best to include and how to make the most of the food choices available to you.

Keeping your kitchen stocked with healthy ingredients is an important part of meal planning and prepping when you have diabetes.

Here are a few suggestions for keeping your kitchen stocked with healthy ingredients:

- **Stock up on whole foods:** Whole foods such as fruits, vegetables, whole grains, lean proteins, and healthy fats, should be the foundation of your diet. Try to have a variety of these items on hand at all times so that you have plenty of options when it comes to meal planning and prepping.

- **Plan your meals**: Before you go to the store, plan your meals for the week. This way, you'll know exactly what ingredients you need and won't be tempted to buy unhealthy items.

- **Buy in bulk:** Buying items such as whole grains, nuts, seeds, and dried fruits in bulk can save money and time.

- **Frozen Foods:** Frozen fruits and vegetables are a great option to have on hand. They are often cheaper than fresh produce, and can be a convenient option when you're short on time.

- **Pantry essentials**: Keep your pantry stocked with essential items such as canned beans, canned tomatoes, and olive oil. These ingredients can be used in a variety of dishes and can help you make a quick meal when you're short on time.

- **Choose lean proteins:** Keep a variety of lean protein options such as chicken, fish, tofu, and eggs in your kitchen. These options are easy to cook and can be a quick meal when you're in a rush.

- **Snack options:** Keep a variety of healthy snack options in your kitchen such as fresh fruits, vegetables, and unsalted nuts.

- **Avoid processed foods:** Try to avoid processed foods as much as possible, as they can be high in added sugars and unhealthy fats.

It's important to keep in mind that everyone's dietary needs are different, so what works for one person may not work for another.

Making the most of leftovers can be a great way to save time, money, and reduce food waste when you have diabetes.

Here are a few suggestions for making the most of leftovers:

- **Plan ahead**: Before cooking a meal, think about how the leftovers could be repurposed for future meals. This way, you can make sure that you're cooking enough food to have leftovers, and you'll know exactly what you'll be using them for.

- **Use different cooking methods:** Leftovers can become unappealing if you eat the same dish multiple times in the same way. Try cooking the leftovers in a different way, such as turning last night's roasted chicken into a stir-fry or making a sandwich out of a previous night's roast beef.

- **Get creative with seasonings**: Leftovers can also become unappealing if you don't mix up the flavors. Experiment with different seasonings, spices, or marinades to give your leftovers a new twist.

- **Utilize your freezer**: If you have more leftovers than you can eat in a few days, consider freezing them. Freezing leftovers in individual portions can make them easy to grab and reheat for a quick and easy meal.

- **Soup it up:** Leftover vegetables can be blended and turned into a delicious and healthy soup. Add some legumes or proteins of your choice and you got yourself a hearty meal.

- **Mix and match**: Leftovers can be combined to create a completely new meal. For example, leftovers from a stir-fry can be mixed with some cooked brown rice and some fresh vegetables for an easy and healthy meal.

- **Repurpose ingredients:** If you have some leftovers that can't be turned into a full meal, use them as ingredients in other dishes. For example, leftover cooked chicken can be diced up and added to a salad, or added to a quesadilla or sandwich.

- **Keep it simple:** Leftovers are easy to prepare, so don't overthink it. Make the most of them with simple methods such as reheating, or turning them into a new dish by adding some ingredients or changing the cooking method.

Maintaining a healthy lifestyle

A healthy lifestyle for people with diabetes goes beyond just food choices and meal planning.

Here are a few additional healthy lifestyle habits to consider:

- **Regular physical activity:** Regular physical activity is important for managing blood sugar levels, maintaining a healthy weight, and reducing the risk of heart disease. Aim for at least 30 minutes of moderate-intensity activity, such as brisk walking, most days of the week.

- **Maintaining a healthy weight**: Maintaining a healthy weight is important for managing diabetes. Losing even a small amount of weight can significantly improve blood sugar control.

- **Stress management:** Stress can affect blood sugar levels, so it's important to manage stress through techniques such as deep breathing, meditation, or yoga.

- **Adequate Sleep**: Getting enough sleep is important for overall health and can help regulate blood sugar levels. Aim for 7-8 hours of sleep per night.

- **Monitoring blood sugar levels:** Keeping track of blood sugar levels can help you manage diabetes and detect any potential issues early on.

- **Regular medical check-ups:** Regular medical check-ups are essential for monitoring diabetes and identifying any potential complications.

- **Quit Smoking** : Smoking can increase the risk of heart disease and other complications in people with diabetes, so quitting smoking is particularly important for people with diabetes.

- **Limit alcohol consumption**: alcohol can affect blood sugar levels, so it's important to limit alcohol consumption and opt for drinks that are lower in carbohydrates, such as wine or light beer.

A collection of delicious and easy-to-prepare recipes that are appropriate for people with diabetes

Here are a few delicious and easy-to-prepare recipe ideas for people with diabetes:

- **Grilled Chicken and Vegetable Skewers**: Thread bite-size pieces of chicken breast and a variety of vegetables, such as bell peppers, onions, and mushrooms, onto skewers. Brush with a marinade made from olive oil, lemon juice, and herbs, and grill until cooked through.

- **Black Bean and Sweet Potato Enchiladas**: Mash cooked sweet potatoes and black beans together with a little bit of diced onion, chili powder, and cumin. Roll this mixture up in corn tortillas and place in a baking dish. Cover with enchilada sauce and shredded cheese, and bake until the cheese is melted and the enchiladas are heated through.

- **Baked Tilapia with Cherry Tomato Salsa**: Mix together diced cherry tomatoes, minced red onion, cilantro, lime juice, and olive oil to make a salsa. Place tilapia filets in a baking dish, and top with the salsa. Bake for 10-12 minutes, or until the fish is cooked through.

- **Cauliflower Fried Rice**: Pulse cauliflower florets in a food processor until they resemble rice. Heat olive oil in a pan, and sauté diced onion and garlic. Add the cauliflower rice, frozen peas, and diced carrots, and sauté until the vegetables are tender. Add beaten eggs, soy sauce, and green onions, and cook until the eggs are set.

- **Vegetable Frittata:** In a skillet saute some chopped vegetables, like bell peppers, onions, spinach, mushroom, etc. Whisk eggs and add them to the skillet. Cook until set and flip to cook the other side.

- **Mediterranean Quinoa Salad**: Cook quinoa according to package instructions and combine it with diced tomatoes, cucumbers, Kalamata olives, feta cheese, and a dressing made from olive oil, lemon juice, and herbs.

- **Turkey and Avocado Lettuce Wraps**: Spread mashed avocado on a lettuce leaf, top it with a few slices of deli turkey, and add any desired toppings such as diced tomatoes, cucumber, bell pepper, or a drizzle of mustard.

- **Spinach and Ricotta Stuffed Chicken Breast**: Stuff chicken breast with a mixture of ricotta cheese, spinach, and herbs. Bake in the oven and topped with a tomato sauce.

- **Grilled Vegetable and Halloumi Skewers:** Cut halloumi cheese and vegetables like bell peppers, onions, and mushrooms and thread them onto skewers. Brush with olive oil and grill until the cheese is browned.

- **Creamy Tomato and Herb Soup**: combine canned tomatoes, chicken or vegetable broth, and herbs such as basil, oregano and thyme and bring to a boil. Reduce heat to low and simmer for 20 minutes. Puree the mixture using an immersion blender or regular blender. Add a touch of cream for extra creaminess.

- **Baked Fish with a Pecan Crust:** Baked Fish with a Pecan Crust is a delicious and healthy recipe that is easy to prepare. Here's a basic recipe that you can follow:

Ingredients:

4 fish fillets (such as salmon or tilapia)

Salt and pepper, to taste

1 cup ground pecans

1/4 cup grated Parmesan cheese

2 tablespoons fresh chopped herbs (such as parsley, basil, or thyme)

2 tablespoons olive oil

Directions:

- ☐ Preheat your oven to 375 degrees F (190 degrees C). Line a baking sheet with parchment paper or lightly oil it.
- ☐ Season the fish fillets with salt and pepper on both sides.
- ☐ In a small bowl, mix together the ground pecans, Parmesan cheese, and herbs.
- ☐ Dip the fish fillets in the olive oil, then coat them with the pecan mixture, pressing it onto the fish to adhere.
- ☐ Place the fish on the prepared baking sheet and bake for 12-15 minutes, or until the fish is cooked through and the crust is golden brown.
- ☐ Serve immediately, garnished with extra herbs if desired.

This recipe can be a good source of omega-3s and protein. Pecans are also a good source of healthy fats and minerals. This recipe is a good way to add variety to your meal plan if you are looking for new ways to cook fish or you are a fish lover.

- **Greek Yogurt Parfait** : Layer Greek yogurt, mixed berries and a drizzle of honey or maple syrup in a cup or jar.

Greek Yogurt Parfait is a delicious and healthy recipe that is easy to prepare. Here's a basic recipe that you can follow:

Ingredients:

2 cups Greek yogurt

1 cup mixed berries (such as strawberries, blueberries, raspberries, etc.)

2 tablespoons honey or maple syrup

1/4 cup granola (optional)

Directions:

- ☐ In a jar or cup, layer 1/4 cup of Greek yogurt at the bottom.
- ☐ Spoon 1/4 cup of mixed berries on top of the yogurt.

☐ Drizzle 1 teaspoon of honey or maple syrup over the berries.

☐ Repeat the layers of yogurt, berries and sweetener until the jar or cup is filled to the top.

☐ Add a sprinkle of granola on top, if desired.

☐ You can also add chopped nuts, seeds or a drizzle of chocolate sauce to make it even more delightful

Note: Greek yogurt is high in protein and calcium, mixed berries are a good source of vitamins, antioxidants, and fiber. Honey or maple syrup add natural sweetness to the dish, instead of using processed sugar. This Greek yogurt parfait can be enjoyed as a breakfast, a snack or a dessert.

- **Brown Rice and Vegetable Stir-fry:** Cook brown rice and stir-fry with your choice of vegetables such as broccoli, peppers, mushrooms, and bok choy. Add a flavorful sauce made from soy sauce, rice vinegar, and sesame oil.

Brown Rice and Vegetable Stir-fry is a delicious and healthy recipe that is easy to prepare. Here's a basic recipe that you can follow:

Ingredients:

1 cup brown rice

2 cups of mixed vegetables (such as broccoli, peppers, mushrooms, and bok choy)

1 tablespoon olive oil

1 tablespoon soy sauce

1 tablespoon rice vinegar

1 teaspoon sesame oil

Salt and pepper, to taste

Directions:

- ☐ Rinse the rice in a fine mesh strainer and add it to a saucepan with 2 cups of water. Bring to a boil, reduce the heat to low, cover and simmer for about 20-25 minutes, or until the rice is cooked.
- ☐ While the rice is cooking, heat the olive oil in a large skillet or wok over medium-high heat.

☐ Add the vegetables and stir-fry for about 5-7 minutes, or until they are tender but still crisp.

☐ In a small bowl, mix together the soy sauce, rice vinegar, and sesame oil.

☐ Once the rice is cooked, add it to the skillet with the vegetables, pour the soy sauce mixture over the top, and stir-fry for another minute or two, until everything is heated through.

☐ Season with salt and pepper, to taste.

☐ Serve hot, garnish with some green onions or sesame seeds if desired.

Note: This recipe can be a good source of fiber and nutrients, brown rice is also a good source of carbohydrates for sustained energy. This recipe is a good way to use up any vegetables that you have on hand and it is a simple, one-pan meal that can be made in under 30 minutes.

- **Brown Rice and Vegetable Stir-Fry:**

☐ Ingredients: 1 cup brown rice, 1 tbsp olive oil, 1 onion, diced, 2 cloves garlic, minced, 2 cups mixed vegetables (such as broccoli, bell peppers, and carrots), 3 tbsp soy sauce, 1 tsp sesame oil

☐ Cook the rice according to package instructions. In a separate pan, heat the olive oil over medium-high heat. Add the onion and garlic and cook until softened. Add the mixed vegetables and stir-fry for 3-4 minutes, or until they are tender. Stir in the cooked rice, soy sauce, and sesame oil.

- **Brown Rice and Black Bean Salad:**

Ingredients: 1 cup brown rice, 1 can black beans, drained and rinsed, 1 red bell pepper, diced, 1/4 cup diced red onion, 2 tbsp lime juice, 2 tbsp olive oil, 1 tsp ground cumin, Salt and pepper

Cook the rice according to package instructions. In a large bowl, combine the cooked rice, black beans, bell pepper, and red onion. In a separate bowl, whisk together the lime juice, olive oil, cumin, salt, and pepper. Pour the dressing over the rice mixture and toss to coat.

- **Brown Rice and Chicken Casserole:**

Ingredients: 1 cup brown rice, 1 lb boneless, skinless chicken breast, diced, 1 onion, diced, 2 cloves garlic, minced, 1 cup frozen mixed vegetables, 1 can diced tomatoes, 1/2 cup grated cheddar cheese.

Cook the rice according to package instructions. Preheat the oven to 375 degrees F. In a separate pan, cook the chicken over medium heat until browned. Add the onion, garlic, and mixed vegetables and cook until softened. Stir in the diced tomatoes and cooked rice. Transfer the mixture to a casserole dish and top with grated cheese. Bake for 20-25 minutes, or until the cheese is melted and bubbly.

Pressing over the quinoa mixture and toss to coat.

- **Quinoa and Vegetable Stir-Fry:**

Ingredients: 1 cup quinoa, 1 tbsp olive oil, 1 onion, diced, 2 cloves garlic, minced, 2 cups mixed vegetables (such as broccoli, bell peppers, and carrots), 3 tbsp soy sauce, 1 tsp sesame oil

Cook the quinoa according to package instructions. In a separate pan, heat the olive oil over medium-high heat.

Add the onion and garlic and cook until softened. Add the mixed vegetables and stir-fry for 3-4 minutes, or until they are tender. Stir in the cooked quinoa, soy sauce, and sesame oil.

- **Quinoa and Chicken Casserole**:

Ingredients: 1 cup quinoa, 1 lb boneless, skinless chicken breast, diced, 1 onion, diced, 2 cloves garlic, minced, 1 cup frozen mixed vegetables, 1 can diced tomatoes, 1/2 cup grated cheddar cheese

Cook the quinoa according to package instructions. Preheat the oven to 375 degrees F. In a separate pan, cook the chicken over medium heat until browned. Add the onion, garlic, and mixed vegetables and cook until softened. Stir in the diced tomatoes and cooked quinoa. Transfer the mixture to a casserole dish and top with grated cheese. Bake for 20-25 minutes, or until the cheese is melted and bubbly.

- **Quinoa and Tuna Salad:**

Ingredients: 1 cup quinoa, 1 can tuna, drained and flaked, 1/4 cup diced red onion, 1/4 cup diced celery, 2 tbsp lemon juice, 2 tbsp mayonnaise, Salt and pepper

Cook the quinoa according to package instructions. In a large bowl, combine the cooked quinoa, tuna, onion, and celery. In a separate bowl, whisk together the lemon juice, mayonnaise, salt, and pepper. Pour the dressing over the quinoa mixture and toss to coat.

- **Quinoa and Roasted Vegetable Salad:**

Ingredients: 1 cup quinoa, 2 cups mixed vegetables (such as bell peppers, zucchini, and eggplant) diced, 2 tbsp olive oil, Salt and pepper, 2 tbsp balsamic vinegar

Cook the quinoa according to package instructions. Preheat the oven to 425 degrees F. In a separate bowl, toss the mixed vegetables with the olive oil, salt and pepper. Roast vegetables in the oven for 15-20 minutes or until tender. In a large bowl, combine the cooked quinoa and roasted vegetables. Toss with balsamic vinaigrette before serving.

- **Quinoa and Black Bean Salad:**

Ingredients: 1 cup quinoa, 1 can black beans, drained and rinsed, 1 red bell pepper, diced, 1/4 cup diced red onion, 2 tbsp lime juice, 2 tbsp olive oil, 1 tsp ground cumin, Salt and pepper

Cook the quinoa according to package instructions. In a large bowl, combine the cooked quinoa, black beans, bell pepper, and red onion. In a separate bowl, whisk together the lime juice, olive oil, cumin, salt, and pepper. Pour the dressing over the quinoa mixture and toss to coat.

- **Whole Wheat French Toast**: Mix together 2 eggs, 1/2 cup of milk, and 1 tsp of vanilla extract. Soak slices of whole wheat bread in the mixture and cook on a griddle until golden brown. Serve with fresh berries and a drizzle of maple syrup.

- **Whole Wheat Grilled Cheese**: Use whole wheat bread and low-fat cheese to make a classic grilled cheese sandwich. Add some tomato or spinach for added flavor and nutrients.

- **Whole Wheat Peanut Butter and Jelly Sandwich:** Spread peanut butter and jelly on whole wheat bread for a tasty and satisfying sandwich. For added protein, you could also add a slice of turkey or ham.

- **Whole Wheat Breakfast Sandwich**: Cook a scrambled egg and some diced turkey bacon. Place the egg and bacon on a whole wheat English muffin with a slice of cheese. This can be a good option for breakfast.

- **Whole Wheat Tuna Salad Sandwich:** Mix canned tuna, diced celery, and a little mayonnaise. Spread the mixture on whole wheat bread and add lettuce and tomato for added flavor and crunch.

- **Whole Wheat Chicken Parmesan Sandwich**: Bread chicken cutlets with whole wheat bread crumbs, and cook until golden brown. Place on a whole wheat roll, top with marinara sauce and mozzarella cheese.

- **Whole Wheat Chicken Caesar Wrap:** Grilled or shredded chicken breast, wrap it with whole wheat tortilla, lettuce, parmesan cheese, and Caesar dressing.

- **Whole Wheat Chicken and Broccoli Casserole:** Mix cooked chicken, steamed broccoli, and a low-fat cream of chicken soup. Place the mixture in a casserole dish, top with whole wheat bread crumbs, and bake until heated through.

- **Whole Wheat Chicken Salad Sandwich:** Mix cooked chicken, diced celery, and a little mayonnaise. Spread the mixture on whole wheat bread and add lettuce and tomato.

- **Whole Wheat Chicken and Vegetable Stir-Fry:** Cook chicken and vegetables of your choice in a stir-fry sauce, and serve over whole wheat rice or noodles.

- **Whole Wheat Chicken and Cheese Quesadilla:** Fill a whole wheat tortilla with shredded chicken, cheese, and vegetables of your choice. Cook on a griddle until the cheese is melted.

- **Whole Wheat Chicken and Mushroom Pie:** Mix cooked chicken and sliced mushrooms with a low-fat cream of mushroom soup. Place the mixture in a pie dish, top with whole wheat pastry crust and bake until heated through.

- **Whole Wheat Chicken and Spinach Souffle:** Mix cooked chicken, spinach, and low-fat cream cheese. Place in a souffle dish and top with whole wheat bread crumbs. Bake until golden brown.

- **Whole Wheat Chicken and Sweet Potato Skillet:** Cook diced chicken and sweet potato in a skillet with your favorite seasonings, and serve with a side of whole wheat bread or crackers.

- **Whole Wheat Chicken and Black Bean Enchiladas**: Fill whole wheat tortillas with a mixture of cooked chicken, black beans, and cheese. Roll them up and place in a baking dish, top with enchilada sauce and cheese, bake until heated through.

- **Baked Chicken and Vegetables:** Mix together diced chicken, vegetables such as bell peppers, zucchini, and tomatoes, olive oil, and your favorite herbs and spices. Place in a baking dish and bake until the chicken is cooked through.

- **Grilled Chicken and Salad**: Grill chicken breast and serve with a salad of mixed greens, tomatoes, cucumbers, and a vinaigrette dressing.

- **Chicken and Mushroom Skillet:** Cook diced chicken and sliced mushrooms in a skillet with olive oil, garlic, and your favorite herbs. Serve with a side of whole grains such as quinoa or brown rice.

- **Chicken and Black Bean Enchiladas**: Fill corn tortillas with a mixture of cooked chicken, black beans, and cheese. Roll them up and place in a baking dish, top with enchilada sauce and cheese, bake until heated through.

- **Chicken and Broccoli Casserole:** Mix together cooked chicken, steamed broccoli, and a low-fat cream of chicken soup. Place the mixture in a casserole dish, top with breadcrumbs and bake until heated through.

- **Chicken and Sweet Potato Curry**: Cook diced chicken and sweet potatoes in a skillet with your choice of curry sauce, and serve with a side of brown rice.

- **Chicken and Green Bean Stir Fry:** Cook chicken and green beans in a skillet with a little olive oil and your favorite stir-fry sauce, and serve with brown rice.

- **Chicken and Quinoa Salad**: Mix cooked chicken, cooked quinoa, mixed greens, tomatoes, and a vinaigrette dressing.

- **Chicken and lentil soup:** Cook diced chicken and lentils in a pot with chicken broth, vegetables such as carrots, celery, and onion, and your choice of herbs and spices.

- **Chicken and Cauliflower Fried Rice :** Make a low carb version of fried rice by replacing white rice with riced cauliflower, mix it with sautéed chicken, vegetables and eggs.

- **Baked Tilapia with herbs and lemon:** Place tilapia fillets on a baking dish and season with herbs such as thyme or rosemary and lemon juice, bake until the fish is cooked through.

- **Grilled Salmon with a side of vegetables:** Season a salmon fillet with your choice of herbs and spices and grill, serve with a side of steamed or grilled vegetables.

- **Pan-Seared Tilapia with a lemon-butter sauce**: Cook tilapia fillets in a skillet with a little olive oil, add butter and lemon juice to make a simple and flavorful sauce.

- **Tuna Salad Lettuce Wraps:** Mix canned tuna with a little mayonnaise and diced celery, wrap it in lettuce leaves for a low-carb alternative to a sandwich.

- **Fish Tacos:** Fill soft corn tortillas with grilled or fried fish, and add your favorite toppings such as shredded cabbage, cilantro and a low-fat yogurt or sour cream.

- **Baked Cod with a Panko Crust:** Coat cod fillets with Panko bread crumbs mixed with herbs and spices, bake until the fish is cooked through.

- **Broiled Halibut with a Tomato-Caper Relish**: Season halibut fillets with herbs and spices, broil, and serve with a relish made from diced tomatoes, capers, and a little olive oil.

- **Fish and Vegetable Curry:** Cook fish fillets in a skillet with your choice of curry sauce and vegetables such as bell peppers and onions. Serve with brown rice or quinoa.

- **Fish Chowder:** Cook diced fish and vegetables such as potatoes, corn and onions, in a pot with chicken or fish broth, add in seasonings such as thyme or dill, and a low-fat milk or cream.

- **Grilled Sardines with a side of Quinoa**: Grill sardines and serve with a side of cooked quinoa and vegetables such as tomato, cucumber, and red onion dressed with a lemon vinaigrette.

- **Tofu Stir Fry:** Cut firm tofu into cubes and stir-fry with your choice of vegetables, such as bell peppers, carrots, and broccoli in a little oil, with your favorite stir-fry sauce.

- **Tofu and Vegetable Curry:** Mix diced tofu and vegetables of your choice in a curry sauce and serve over brown rice or quinoa.

- **Tofu Scramble:** Crumble firm tofu into a pan and cook with your choice of vegetables such as bell peppers and onion, season with turmeric and nutritional yeast for a vegan version of scrambled eggs.

- **Tofu and Vegetable Skewers:** Cut firm tofu into cubes and vegetables such as bell peppers, zucchini, and mushrooms, marinate in a little olive oil, soy sauce, and your favorite herbs and spices, and grill or broil.

- **Tofu and Eggplant Casserole:** Mix diced tofu and eggplant with a little olive oil, tamari, and herbs, bake in a casserole dish until heated through.

- **Tofu and vegetable Spring rolls :** Mix diced tofu, shredded vegetables such as carrots, cucumber and cabbage with a little soy sauce, rice vinegar and ginger, wrap it in rice paper or spring roll wrapper and deep fry.

- **Tofu and Broccoli Stir Fry**: Cut tofu into cubes and stir-fry with broccoli florets in a little oil, with your choice of seasonings such as ginger and garlic.

- **Tofu and Mushroom Stroganoff:** Cook sliced mushrooms and crumbled tofu in a skillet with a little flour, vegetable broth, and a non-dairy cream, serve over whole wheat pasta.

- **Tofu and Kale Salad**: Mix cubed tofu and torn kale with diced vegetables such as bell peppers and cherry tomatoes, dress with a vinaigrette made from olive oil and lemon juice.

- **Tofu and Vegetable Curry Soup:** Mix diced tofu and vegetables with your choice of curry powder, coconut milk and vegetable broth and simmer until heated through.

- **Egg and Vegetable Omelette:** Whisk together eggs, diced vegetables such as bell peppers, mushrooms, and onions, and a little milk or cream, pour into a hot skillet and cook until set.

- **Egg and Turkey Bacon Breakfast Sandwich**: Cook an egg and a slice of turkey bacon, place on a whole wheat English muffin with a slice of cheese.

- **Egg and Vegetable Frittata:** Whisk together eggs, diced vegetables, and a little milk or cream, pour into a hot skillet and cook until set, then transfer to the oven and bake until fully cooked.

- **Egg and Avocado Toast:** Mash avocado on whole wheat toast and top with a fried or poached egg.

- **Egg and Tomato Salad**: Mix hard-boiled eggs with diced tomatoes, cucumbers, and a vinaigrette dressing.

- **Egg and Mushroom Scramble**: Cook diced mushrooms and crumbled turkey bacon with scrambled eggs, season with herbs such as chives or parsley.

- **Egg and Spinach Quiche:** Mix together eggs, spinach, low-fat milk, and a little grated cheese, pour into a whole wheat pie crust and bake until set.

- **Egg and Ham Breakfast Burrito:** Scramble eggs and diced ham and wrap them in a whole wheat tortilla, with veggies and cheese of your choice.

- **Egg and Broccoli Fried Rice:** Use leftover brown rice, sautéed broccoli and eggs to make a low-carb version of fried rice.

- **Egg and Sardine Salad:** Mix flaked canned sardines with chopped hard-boiled eggs, celery and a little mayonnaise, serve on a bed of greens or as a sandwich.

- **Spinach and Feta Omelette:** Whisk together eggs, baby spinach, and crumbled feta cheese, cook in a skillet until set.

- **Kale and Quinoa Salad:** Mix cooked quinoa, diced vegetables, and torn kale leaves, dress with a vinaigrette made from olive oil and lemon juice.

- **Green Smoothie:** Blend spinach, kale, or other leafy greens with a little fruit and a liquid such as almond milk or yogurt, and you can add a scoop of protein powder to make it more nutritious

- **Arugula and Tomato Salad:** Mix arugula leaves with diced tomatoes, cucumbers, and a vinaigrette dressing.

- **Spinach and Feta Stuffed Chicken Breast:** Roll boneless chicken breast with a mixture of spinach and feta cheese, season, and bake until fully cooked.

- **Collard Greens and Black-eyed peas:** Cook collard greens with diced onions, garlic and smoked turkey or ham hocks for the traditional southern way.

- **Spinach and Mushroom Quiche:** Mix together eggs, spinach, sliced mushrooms, low-fat milk, and a little grated cheese, pour into a whole wheat pie crust and bake until set.

- **Bok Choy and Sesame Chicken Stir Fry:** Stir-fry sliced bok choy with diced chicken and your choice of stir-fry sauce, serve with sesame seeds and brown rice.

- **Kale Chips:** Toss kale leaves with a little olive oil and seasonings of your choice, then bake in the oven until crispy.

- **Spinach and Artichoke Dip:** Mix together chopped spinach, canned artichoke hearts, low-fat cream cheese, and grated Parmesan cheese, bake until heated through and serve with whole wheat crackers or vegetables for dipping.

- **Broccoli and Cheddar Soup:** Cook chopped broccoli in a pot with chicken or vegetable broth and a little milk or cream, blend until smooth and stir in grated cheddar cheese until melted.

- **Broccoli and Chicken Stir Fry:** Stir fry diced chicken and broccoli florets in a little oil with your favorite stir-fry sauce, serve over brown rice.

- **Broccoli and Quinoa Salad:** Mix cooked quinoa, diced vegetables, and chopped broccoli, dress with a vinaigrette made from olive oil and lemon juice.

- **Broccoli and Cheddar Casserole:** Mix together cooked broccoli and a low-fat cheddar cheese sauce, top with breadcrumbs and bake until heated through.

- **Broccoli and Tofu Stir Fry:** Stir fry diced tofu and broccoli florets in a little oil with your favorite stir-fry sauce, serve over brown rice or quinoa.

- **Broccoli and Parmesan Fritters:** Mix together grated broccoli, eggs, grated Parmesan cheese, and flour, form into patties and fry in a little oil until golden brown.

- **Broccoli and Cauliflower Cream Soup :** Cook diced broccoli and cauliflower in a pot with chicken or vegetable broth, puree and stir in a low-fat cream to make it creamy.

- **Broccoli and egg salad:** Boil eggs, mix them with diced broccoli, chopped celery and a low-fat mayonnaise, season with black pepper.

- **Broccoli and shrimp stir fry**: stir fry shrimp, broccoli florets and other vegetables with garlic and your favorite stir-fry sauce.

- **Broccoli and Parmesan Risotto :** Cook Arborio rice with a low-fat broth, diced broccoli and grated Parmesan cheese to make a creamy and healthy risotto.

- **Bell Pepper and Feta Omelette**: A high-protein breakfast option that's easy to make and packed with flavor.

Ingredients:
2 large bell peppers (red, yellow or green), diced
1/4 cup crumbled feta cheese
4 large eggs
Salt and pepper, to taste
2 teaspoons olive oil

Optional: chopped herbs like parsley or chives for garnish

Instructions:
- ☐ Heat a medium non-stick skillet over medium heat.
- ☐ Add the olive oil to the skillet.
- ☐ Once the oil is hot, add the diced bell peppers to the skillet and sauté for about 5 minutes or until they are softened.
- ☐ In a bowl, whisk the eggs, salt and pepper together.
- ☐ Pour the eggs over the bell peppers and cook for about 1-2 minutes until the bottom of the omelette is set.
- ☐ Sprinkle feta cheese on one half of the omelette and then use a spatula to fold the other half over the feta cheese.
- ☐ Cook the omelette for 1-2 minutes or until the cheese is melted and the eggs are set.
- ☐ Carefully slide the omelette onto a plate, garnish with chopped herbs if desired.

This is a balanced meal that includes protein, healthy fats, and vegetables. You can serve it with a side salad or roasted vegetables if you like, but it's also a filling meal on its own.

- **Stuffed Bell Peppers**: A classic dish that can be filled with a variety of healthy ingredients, such as ground turkey, quinoa, or brown rice.

Ingredients:

4 large bell peppers (red, yellow or green), halved and seeded

1 pound lean ground turkey or beef

1 cup cooked quinoa or brown rice

1/2 cup diced tomatoes

1/2 cup diced onions

1/2 cup diced mushrooms

1/2 cup diced bell peppers

2 cloves of garlic, minced

1 teaspoon olive oil

Salt and pepper, to taste

1 cup grated cheese (optional)

Instructions:

- ☐ Preheat the oven to 375°F (190°C).
- ☐ In a large skillet, heat the olive oil over medium heat.
- ☐ Add the ground turkey or beef, and cook until browned. Drain off any excess fat.
- ☐ Add the onions, mushrooms, bell peppers, and garlic to the skillet and cook for 5 minutes or until softened.
- ☐ Stir in the diced tomatoes, salt, pepper, quinoa or rice and mix well.
- ☐ Place the bell pepper halves in a baking dish, and fill each one with the turkey or beef mixture.
- ☐ If desired, top each bell pepper with grated cheese.
- ☐ Cover the baking dish with aluminum foil and bake for 30-35 minutes or until the bell peppers are tender.
- ☐ Remove the foil and bake for an additional 10 minutes or until the cheese is melted and bubbly.
- ☐ Let cool for a few minutes before serving.

Note: This recipe is packed with vegetables and lean protein, making it a healthy and satisfying meal. To make it more diabetic friendly you can adjust the quantity of cheese or even leave it out. Also, you can use a smaller portion size, or even more veggies to reduce the carb content.

- **Grilled Bell Pepper Salad:** A simple and refreshing salad that pairs well with a variety of proteins.

Ingredients:
2 large bell peppers, (red, yellow or green) sliced
1 large red onion, sliced
2 cloves of garlic, minced
2 tablespoons olive oil
Salt and pepper, to taste
2 tablespoons red wine vinegar
2 tablespoons fresh lemon juice
2 tablespoons chopped fresh basil or parsley
Optional: add protein like grilled chicken or shrimp

Instructions:
- ☐ Preheat the grill to medium-high heat.
- ☐ In a small bowl, mix together the olive oil, garlic, salt, and pepper.

☐ Toss the sliced bell peppers and red onion with the olive oil mixture.

☐ Grill the bell peppers and onions for about 8-10 minutes or until they are slightly charred and tender.

☐ In a large bowl, whisk together the red wine vinegar, lemon juice, salt and pepper.

☐ Once the vegetables are cooked, add them to the large bowl and toss to coat with the dressing.

☐ Top with fresh herbs and any protein if desired.

Note: This recipe is low in carbohydrates, high in fiber and vitamins from the bell peppers, and a good source of healthy fats from the olive oil. To further tailor the recipe to your needs, you can adjust the quantity of the dressing or leave out any proteins if it's not necessary.

- Bell Pepper and Black Bean Tacos: A tasty and satisfying vegetarian option that's high in fiber and protein.

Ingredients:

1 tablespoon olive oil

1 medium onion, diced

2 cloves of garlic, minced

1 red bell pepper, diced

1 yellow bell pepper, diced

1 cup of cooked black beans

1 teaspoon ground cumin

1 teaspoon chili powder

Salt and pepper, to taste

8 corn tortillas

1/4 cup of crumbled feta cheese

1/4 cup of chopped cilantro

Lime wedges, for serving

Instructions:

- ☐ Heat the olive oil in a large skillet over medium heat. Add the onion and garlic and sauté for about 3 minutes.
- ☐ Add the diced bell peppers and cook for an additional 5 minutes.
- ☐ Add the black beans, cumin, chili powder, salt, and pepper to the skillet. Cook for an additional 2-3 minutes until everything is heated through.
- ☐ While the pepper and beans are cooking, warm the corn tortillas in the oven or on a skillet.

☐ To assemble the tacos, place a few spoonfuls of the pepper and bean mixture in the center of each warm tortilla.

☐ Top with crumbled feta cheese and chopped cilantro.

☐ Serve with lime wedges.

Some things to keep in mind:

I.   Avoid adding extra sugar or honey to the dish, as it is high in carbohydrate.

II. Use cheese, sour cream or avocado to add some healthy fat instead.

III. Using corn tortillas will give you some extra fiber and lower the glycemic index of the meal.

- **Bell Pepper and Chicken Stir-Fry:** A quick and easy way to get in a serving of vegetables with a lean protein source.

Ingredients:

1 pound boneless, skinless chicken breasts, cut into thin strips

2 red bell peppers, sliced

2 green bell peppers, sliced

2 tablespoons olive oil

2 cloves garlic, minced

2 tablespoons low-sodium soy sauce

1 teaspoon cornstarch

1 teaspoon sesame oil

1 teaspoon honey (Optional)

salt and pepper, to taste

Instructions:

- ☐ Heat the olive oil in a large skillet or wok over high heat.
- ☐ Add the chicken and stir-fry for 5-6 minutes, or until cooked through. Remove from skillet and set aside.
- ☐ Add bell peppers to skillet and stir-fry for 3-4 minutes, or until they begin to soften.
- ☐ Add garlic and stir-fry for 1 more minute.
- ☐ In a small bowl, mix together the soy sauce, cornstarch, sesame oil, honey (if using) and some salt and pepper.
- ☐ Add the sauce to the skillet and stir-fry until the sauce thickens, about 1-2 minutes.

☐ Add the chicken back to the skillet and stir-fry until the chicken is heated through and the vegetables are coated in the sauce.

☐ Serve over rice or noodles and enjoy!

Note: The honey is optional, it is only there to add more sweetness but you can skip it to make it a lower carb dish. You can also experiment with other veggies or even tofu as protein sources.

Adjust seasoning to taste and also you can check for salt or soy sauce with your doctor or dietary specialist to make sure it's okay for your individual situation.

- **Bell Pepper and Tomato Soup**: A comforting and flavorful soup that's easy to make in a large batch and reheat throughout the week.

Ingredients:

2 tbsp olive oil

1 onion, diced

2 cloves garlic, minced

2 bell peppers (red or yellow), diced

3 cups fresh tomatoes, diced

4 cups low-sodium chicken or vegetable broth

1 tsp dried basil

Salt and pepper, to taste

Stevia or Erythritol or any sugar alternative to taste

Directions:

- ☐ Heat the olive oil in a large pot over medium heat. Add the onion, garlic, and bell peppers, and sauté for about 5 minutes, until the vegetables are softened.
- ☐ Add the diced tomatoes, broth, basil, and salt and pepper, and bring the soup to a simmer.
- ☐ Simmer for about 20 minutes, or until the vegetables are tender.
- ☐ Season with stevia or any sugar alternative to taste.
- ☐ Puree the soup with a blender until smooth, or use an immersion blender directly in the pot.
- ☐ Serve the soup hot, and garnish with chopped fresh basil or parsley, if desired.
- ☐ You can make it a full meal by serving it with a side of greens or salads and some low-carb crackers.

- **Bell Pepper and Mushroom Risotto**: A creamy and satisfying dish that's perfect for a special occasion or a cozy night in.

Ingredients:

1 tablespoon olive oil

1 onion, diced

2 cloves garlic, minced

8 ounces sliced mushrooms

1 red bell pepper, diced

1 green bell pepper, diced

1 cup Arborio rice

3 cups chicken or vegetable broth, low-sodium

1/2 cup grated Parmesan cheese

2 tablespoons chopped fresh parsley

Salt and pepper, to taste

Instructions:

- ☐ Heat the olive oil in a large skillet over medium heat.
- ☐ Add the onion and garlic and cook until softened, about 5 minutes.

- ☐ Add the mushrooms, red bell pepper and green bell pepper, and cook for another 5-7 minutes, or until the vegetables are tender.
- ☐ Add the rice to the skillet and stir until the rice is well coated and beginning to turn translucent, about 1-2 minutes.
- ☐ Slowly pour in the broth, one ladleful at a time, stirring constantly. Wait until the liquid is absorbed before adding the next ladleful.
- ☐ Continue to cook and stir until the rice is tender and the risotto is creamy, about 20-25 minutes.
- ☐ Stir in the Parmesan cheese and parsley.
- ☐ Season to taste with salt and pepper.
- ☐ Serve in bowls and enjoy!

Note: You can use other kind of cheese or even use less cheese as per your dietary restriction. Also, It's best to use homemade broth instead of store-bought, as it is lower in sodium.

Bell Pepper and Zucchini Noodles: A low-carb and gluten-free alternative to traditional pasta dishes.

Ingredients:

2 medium zucchinis

2 bell peppers (any color), thinly sliced

2 cloves of garlic, minced

2 tablespoons olive oil

Salt and pepper, to taste

Optional: grated Parmesan cheese or chopped fresh herbs for serving

Instructions:

- [ ] Use a spiralizer, julienne peeler, or a sharp knife to create noodles from the zucchinis.
- [ ] In a large pan, heat the olive oil over medium heat. Add the garlic and sauté for 30 seconds, until fragrant.
- [ ] Add the bell pepper and sauté for about 5 minutes, or until tender.
- [ ] Add the zucchini noodles and sauté for 2-3 minutes, or until the noodles are cooked to your liking. Be careful not to overcook the noodles as they will become mushy.
- [ ] Season with salt and pepper to taste.
- [ ] Serve immediately, topped with grated Parmesan cheese or chopped fresh herbs if desired.

☐ It is very easy to cook, healthy and low on carbohydrate which is best for diabetes patients.

- **Bell Pepper and Eggplant Parmesan**: A lighter version of a classic Italian dish that's just as flavorful and satisfying.

Ingredients:

1 medium eggplant, sliced into 1/4-inch rounds

1 red bell pepper, sliced

1 yellow bell pepper, sliced

1/2 cup all-purpose flour

2 eggs, beaten

1 cup whole wheat bread crumbs

1/4 cup grated Parmesan cheese

Salt and pepper, to taste

2 cups marinara sauce

1 cup shredded mozzarella cheese

Instructions:

☐ Preheat the oven to 375 degrees F (190 degrees C). Grease a baking sheet or line with parchment paper.

- ☐ In a shallow dish, combine the flour, salt, and pepper. In another shallow dish, place the beaten eggs. In a third shallow dish, combine the bread crumbs and grated Parmesan cheese.
- ☐ Dip the eggplant and bell pepper slices in the flour mixture, then the eggs, and finally the bread crumb mixture. Place the coated slices on the prepared baking sheet.
- ☐ Bake for 20-25 minutes, or until the eggplant and bell pepper slices are golden brown and tender.
- ☐ In a 9x13 inch baking dish, spread a thin layer of marinara sauce on the bottom of the dish. Layer the baked eggplant and bell pepper slices on top of the sauce. Pour the remaining marinara sauce over the eggplant and bell pepper slices, and sprinkle the shredded mozzarella cheese on top.
- ☐ Bake in the preheated oven for an additional 20-25 minutes, or until the cheese is melted and bubbly. Let the dish cool for a few minutes before serving.

Note: You can add or replace with other vegetables as well according to your taste.

It's good to consume after its cooled down and can be served with whole wheat pasta or bread.

Bell Pepper and Lentil Curry: A hearty and flavorful dish that's perfect for a cold winter day.

www.ingramcontent.com/pod-product-compliance
Lightning Source LLC
Chambersburg PA
CBHW071550260726
48653CB00007BA/2641